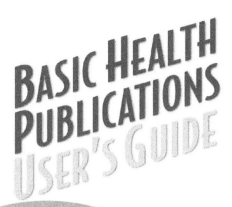

BASIC HEALTH
PUBLICATIONS
USER'S GUIDE

TO
VITAMIN E

*Don't Be a Dummy.
Become an Expert
on What Vitamin E
Can Do for Your
Health.*

JACK CHALLEM &
MELISSA DIANE SMITH
JACK CHALLEM Series Editor

Series Editor: Jack Challem
Editor: Roberta W. Waddell
Typesetter: Gary A. Rosenberg
Series Cover Designer: Mike Stromberg

Basic Health Publications User's Guides are published by Basic Health Publications, Inc.

CONTENTS

INTRODUCTION

Could one single vitamin reduce your risk of developing heart disease, cancer, and Alzheimer's disease?

If the supplement is vitamin E, the answer is yes. Does this sound too incredible to be true? Read on, and you may change your mind.

Discovered in 1922, vitamin E was for years the butt of jokes that referred to it disparagingly as the sex vitamin. Amazingly, as far back as the 1940s, a team of Canadian physicians discovered that vitamin E could protect people from coronary heart disease. But because these doctors could not explain, in scientific terms, why vitamin E worked, they were dismissed as quacks and charlatans. And for many years to come, vitamin E would be regarded as a "cure in search of a disease" and nothing more than a waste of money.

Fast-forward to the present, and the view of vitamin E is strikingly different. Scientific research has caught up with this remarkable nutrient. Today, with thousands of studies to support it, vitamin E is quickly being recognized as the closest thing to a "magic bullet" in the prevention of Alzheimer's disease, cancer, heart disease, and many other disorders.

So, what exactly makes vitamin E so great? Scientists tell us that age-related diseases—and the risk of most diseases increases with age—are caused in part by hazardous molecules known as free radicals. Free radicals make iron rust and butter turn rancid. In a sense, they make your body more rusty and rancid with age.

Nature, however, provided a way to neutralize free radicals—with a group of beneficial molecules called antioxidants. Vitamin E stands out as one of the most powerful antioxidants found in foods. It scavenges free radicals in the body and limits their damage. In so doing, vitamin E slows the aging process and reduces the long-term risk of age-related degenerative diseases. It doesn't matter if you're a woman or a man—vitamin E can provide all people with important health benefits.

But, you might be wondering, don't we all get enough vitamin E in the foods we eat? And if vitamin E is so great, why don't doctors recommend it?

Over the past century, the Western diet has undergone tremendous changes. The foods most people eat are highly processed, and vitamin E (along with many other nutrients) is removed. The typical American is consuming only a small percentage of the vitamin E his or her grandparents consumed.

In addition, our nutritional requirements for vitamin E have increased. Most people are eating more fried foods and vegetable oil than people consumed in the past. These foods are prone to free radical damage and boost our need for vit-amin E. Also, with more industrialization and the increased use of polluting automobiles, people have been exposed to unprecedented levels of air pollution. This also boosts our need for vita-min E.

As for doctors, they have slowly but steadily

been catching on to the benefits of vitamin E. In recent years, the scientific research on this amazing nutrient has become an irresistible force in medicine. One recent survey found that almost half of all cardiologists were taking vitamin E supplements themselves, though they were a bit reluctant to recommend them to patients. When we ask physicians about vitamin E, they say that nearly every doctor takes the vitamin.

The question, now, might be this: Why aren't you taking vitamin E?

In this *User's Guide to Vitamin E*, we will tell you about the remarkable story of vitamin E and how it can reduce your risk of serious, degenerative diseases and how it may even help protect you against infections. First, in Chapter 1 we will explain how vitamin E prevents heart disease, the leading cause of death among Americans and most other Westerners. In Chapter 2, we'll describe the exciting research showing that vitamin E can probably reduce your long-term risk of cancer, including breast cancer in women and prostate cancer in men. Later in this book, we'll cover how vitamin E can protect you from numerous other diseases, including Alzheimer's and additional neurological disorders, cataracts, infertility, and menopausal hot flashes. Lastly, in Chapter 8, we'll explain how to shop for the best types of vitamin E which, according to research, are the natural forms of this vitamin.

CHAPTER 1

PROTECTING THE HEART

Heart disease is the leading cause of death among men and women in most Western nations. It has killed more Americans than all wars combined. Heart disease is complex and develops subtly and slowly. It has multiple causes, but a lack of vitamin E is paramount among the reasons it develops. In this chapter, we'll look at the causes of heart disease, some different aspects of this condition, and the many ways vitamin E helps prevent heart disease.

Vitamin E Reduces the Risk of Heart Disease

Research and the clinical experiences of physicians show beyond a doubt that vitamin E is good for the heart. Evidence supporting the role of vitamin E as a heart protector has been building for decades. In the past several years, the evidence has become so strong that most doctors can't ignore it.

For example, Harvard University researchers reported in the *New England Journal of Medicine* that vitamin E supplements dramatically reduced the risk of coronary heart disease in men and women. The amount of vitamin E used—more than 100 IU (international units)—was more than six times the Recommended Dietary Allowance

(RDA) for vitamin E. This is an amount you can obtain only from supplements, not foods.

Even more impressive were the results of a blockbuster study reported in the British medical journal *Lancet*. Researchers from the University of Cambridge in England gave either 400 or 800 IU of natural vitamin E or placebos (dummy pills) daily to 2,000 patients with confirmed heart disease. The group taking vitamin E for an average of eighteen months had a remarkable 77 percent lower incidence of nonfatal heart attacks compared to the placebo group.

Those British researchers pronounced vitamin E more powerful in controlling heart attacks than aspirin or cholesterol-lowering drugs—and the benefits of vitamin E were evident within only six and one-half months after the subjects started taking it. So impressive were these results that the American Heart Association ranked vitamin E number four on its list of the top ten heart-related developments in 1996.

Vitamin E
The body's principal fat-soluble antioxidant that is incorporated into cell membranes and protects cells from free radical damage.

The encouraging research results with vitamin E for heart health continue. In an analysis of the five largest trials investigating vitamin E for heart health, published in the journal *Current Opinion in Lipidology*, the authors concluded that alpha-tocopherol (the most common form of vitamin E) was beneficial in patients with pre-existing heart disease. In the majority of these studies, those taking the alpha-tocopherol supplements had a reduced risk of a nonfatal heart attack. The one study of the five showing no benefit was criticized for its poor design.

Additional recent research, also published in

Lancet, has found that vitamin E helps prevent heart disease in kidney dialysis patients who are four times more likely to die of cardiovascular disease than healthy people. In the study, a dose of 800 IU of natural vitamin E or a placebo daily for an average of seventeen months was given to dialysis patients. Seventeen patients who took placebos had heart attacks during the study, but only five of the patients who took vitamin E had heart attacks during the study.

Occasionally you'll hear that a new study has found no protective effect of vitamin E on heart health or some other condition. That's a good time to take a critical look at the study's design. For how long did the subjects take vitamin E to gauge results? You probably need to take vitamin E for years to experience long-term benefits. Also, was natural vitamin E (far superior to synthetic) used in the study? Sadly, many published studies still don't even distinguish whether the natural or synthetic form was used. Yet these questions—even if they go unanswered in your search for information—highlight just a couple of the factors that affect research outcomes.

Understanding the Vitamin E Connection to Heart Health

It may be hard to believe, but it has been more than half a century since doctors first discovered that vitamin E could prevent heart disease. In the 1940s, Evan Shute, M.D., and his colleagues in London, Canada, reported that vitamin E could reverse many symptoms of heart disease. Although their findings were described in 1946 in the respected scientific journal *Nature,* as well as in *Time* magazine, the medical establishment largely rejected their findings.

Part of the reason was that most doctors at the time could not imagine how a mere vitamin would protect against the leading cause of death among Americans and Canadians. Over the years, vitamin E was ridiculed. Some people considered it a waste of money; others called it "a cure in search of a disease."

During the 1980s and 1990s, researchers quietly built a strong scientific case to support vitamin E. Simply put, vitamin E is a protective substance called an antioxidant. It neutralizes harmful substances called oxidants, or free radicals. During this time, the free radical theory of aging—and age-related diseases—gained momentum as well. So, as an antioxidant, vitamin E could be considered an antiaging and antidisease vitamin. The human studies of the 1990s clearly demonstrated its benefits—and proved Shute correct in his original observations that vitamin E was good for the heart.

Free radicals are molecules that have one unpaired electron. As a consequence, they're highly unstable. In an effort to become more stable, free radicals cruise around inside the body, aggressively seeking compounds with which they can react to gain an electron. They can damage anything they come across—fats, sugars, your cells and the DNA inside your cells, to name a few—in the process.

Free Radicals
Harmful molecules produced by the body and pollutants. They have one electron too few or one too many, making them highly unstable.

Antioxidants quench free radicals by donating electrons to make up for the missing ones in free radicals. This means that antioxidants scavenge free radicals before they cause harm to our cells. Think of antioxidants as bodyguards that protect cells from damage by free radicals. This kind of damage is implicated in the development and spread of not just heart disease but all degenerative diseases, as you'll read many times throughout this book. Taking antioxidants such as vitamin E is important for protecting the whole body—not just the heart—against disease.

How Heart Disease Develops

Heart disease (sometimes referred to as coronary artery disease) develops slowly, usually without our knowledge, in a step-by-step progression of events. It begins when artery walls become damaged or injured by free radicals. "Smooth muscle cells" then begin to grow on artery walls and plaque forms.

Then a series of events occurs that cause artery walls to become clogged with fat and cholesterol. If the artery walls become too narrow and if the blood becomes sticky and blood clots form, blood flow can become restricted. Blood clots in arteries are sort of like a wad of hair caught in a drainpipe; blood (or water, in your bathroom sink) can't get past the blockage to where it's supposed to go.

When blood flow is restricted, the heart doesn't receive the oxygen from blood that it needs to function. The result can be a heart attack or stroke. Heart tissue dies as a result of the blood supply being cut off (as in a heart attack), making the heart weaker. A heart attack can disrupt the heartbeat, which is controlled by rhythmic electrical activity within the heart itself. The most common form of stroke is called ischemic stroke, which results from decreased blood supply to the brain and leads to neurological problems. Often, a stroke is caused by cholesterol-containing deposits of plaque which block blood flow in the arteries supplying the brain.

Vitamin E, as an antioxidant, protects both the artery walls and the cholesterol found in our bloodstream from free radical damage. Both of these protections help prevent heart disease from developing and progressing. And, considering the serious consequences of this major killer, that's very good news.

Vitamin E's Protective Effects on Cholesterol

In discussing heart health, many people wonder how cholesterol is affected. Vitamin E won't actually lower high blood levels of cholesterol, but it does protect against heart disease by doing something more important—it prevents the low-density lipoprotein (LDL) form of cholesterol from being chemically changed and becoming toxic to arteries. LDL cholesterol is often referred to as "bad" cholesterol, but it isn't inherently bad. Low levels of LDL are actually needed to transport vitamin E and other fat-soluble vitamins through the bloodstream.

LDL becomes harmful to arteries when there is insufficient vitamin E in our system to prevent it from being oxidized, or damaged, by free radicals. This damage is called lipid peroxidation. Without enough antioxidants, circulating free radicals in the body damage the structure of LDL, making it appear foreign to the immune system. This system, attempting to protect us from foreign invaders, sends out immune cells to engulf the oxidized LDL.

These immune cells filled with lipids, called foam cells, clump together on blood vessel surfaces. This is plaque, which then builds up, limiting the flow of oxygen and other nutrients in the blood to the heart. Avoiding LDL oxidation is one of the central goals in current preventive and therapeutic natural approaches to staving off heart disease. Studies in animals and humans consistently show that 400–500 IU of vitamin

LDLs
Low-density lipoproteins, which transport proteins, triglycerides (fats), cholesterol and fat-soluble vitamins through the blood to body cells.

E daily protects LDL from oxidation, thus preventing LDL deposits in blood vessels and reducing the risk of coronary heart disease.

In one such study, published in the journal *Arteriosclerosis, Thrombosis, and Vascular Biology*, forty-eight men and women aged forty-five to sixty-nine took either 271 IU of natural vitamin E, 500 mg of vitamin C, a combination of the two, or a placebo daily for three years. Both vitamin E and the combination of vitamins C and E made the LDL cholesterol in these men and women less prone to oxidation. (Vitamin C alone had no effect.) Another recent study found that people with coronary heart disease who took 400 IU of vitamin E per day for thirty days had significant decreases in lipid peroxidation compared to a placebo group. Others taking vitamin C, vitamin A, or increasing their fruit intake also experienced decreased oxidative damage, but not as much as the vitamin E group did.

If you take cholesterol-lowering drugs, it's especially important for you to take vitamin E. These drugs cause vitamin E levels in LDL to drop and LDL, in turn, oxidizes more quickly than normal. Thus, although such drugs do lower cho - lesterol levels, they may actually increase the damage to blood vessel walls. (Supplementing with the vitaminlike antioxidant coenzyme Q_{10} is also a good idea for people taking cholesterol-lowering drugs.)

Vitamin E's Other Heart-Protective Benefits

Vitamin E works in a variety of ways beyond that of an antioxidant to slow or stop the development of heart disease and stroke. As you've read, it slows down the buildup of smooth muscle cells on artery walls that contribute to artery-clogging plaque. In some people, vitamin E also may increase levels of the high-density lipoprotein (HDL) form of cholesterol, the type that is called the "good" cholesterol because it carries cholesterol from the bloodstream to the liver for elimination.

> **Platelet Aggregation**
> *The tendency of blood platelets to stick together, promoting blood clot formation.*

Vitamin E decreases excessive platelet aggregation, too. This is the tendency of blood platelets to stick together and promote the formation of blood clots, which increase the risk of heart attack and stroke because they restrict blood flow. The blood-thinning benefits of vitamin E make it particularly important for those with diabetes and women who take oral contraceptives, because these groups have an increased tendency for excessive platelet aggregation and higher risk of stroke.

In a recent study, Jane E. Freedman, M.D., and John F. Keaney, M.D., found that natural vitamin E was well absorbed by blood platelets in blood taken from healthy volunteers. The synthetic form was not well absorbed (you'll learn more about the advantages of natural over synthetic vitamin E in Chapter 8). The researchers determined that natural vitamin E reduced platelet aggregation by more than half! In other research, published in the journal *Atherosclerosis, Thrombosis, and Vascular Biology*, vitamin E supplements taken daily for two weeks decreased platelet aggregation and led to lower levels of free radicals in human subjects.

Keep in mind that reducing platelet aggregation, or stickiness, decreases the likelihood of blood clots and a resulting cardiac event. Interestingly, Freedman and Keaney found that the anticoagulant effect of vitamin E was not related to its antioxidant properties. Rather, it was because vitamin E inhibits protein kinase C, an enzyme that promotes blood clotting and breakdown of collagen tissue.

Vitamin E Protects against the Harmful Effects of Junk Foods

According to recent studies, vitamin E can even protect you from some of the cardiovascular effects of high-fat/high-carbohydrate foods—a combination found in most convenience, microwave, and "fast" foods. Fatty meals normally trigger a chain of chemical reactions that tense up, or constrict, blood vessels, leading to reduced blood flow. This cardiovascular consequence is called endothelial dysfunction. A fascinating study by cardiologist Gary Plotnick, M.D., of the University of Maryland, found that vitamin E and vitamin C offer significant protection against the damaging effects of high-fat/high-carbohydrate meals.

In the study, twenty faculty members ate a popular, high-fat, fast-food breakfast consisting of

Endothelial Dysfunction

A pronounced constriction of blood vessels that leads to a stiffening of blood-vessel walls and reduced blood flow, increasing the risk of heart disease.

eggs and sausage on a roll along with hash browns. As the researchers expected, the fat burden of this breakfast prevented the subjects' arteries from relaxing, or dilating, normally. Normal dilation is necessary for normal blood flow.

On another day, the same subjects ate the same breakfast, but about fifteen minutes before eating they also took 800 IU of vitamin E and 1,000 mg vitamin C. This combination offered remarkable protection. Their blood vessels behaved normally, as if they had eaten low-fat foods—and the benefits lasted for six hours.

Unfortunately, Plotnick blamed the endothelial dysfunction only on what he described as a meal high in saturated fat. While the fast-food breakfast was high in saturated fat, it was also high in hydrogenated vegetable oils, trans fatty acids (now known to be much worse than saturated fat), oxidized fats, and refined carbohydrates. So, rather than just being an indictment of saturated fats, Plotnick actually showed the overall danger of a typical fast-food meal—and how vitamins E and C could blunt part of the damage.

Another study, conducted by David L. Katz, M.D., and his colleagues at the Yale University School of Medicine, echoed these findings. Fifty healthy, nonsmoking men and women had decreased blood flow in their forearms after drinking a milkshake made with ice cream, coconut cream and pasteurized eggs—a high-fat (and high-sugar) meal. On separate occasions, these same subjects were given—individually—either 800 IU of vitamin E in capsule form, oatmeal, or whole-wheat cereal, in addition to the milkshake. The vitamin E supplements and the oatmeal (independently) protected against any reduction in blood flow.

Once again, this researcher conducted a study that attempted to show the cardiovascular effects of a high-fat meal. But, in actuality, he demonstrated the hazards of a high-fat/high-carbohydrate meal because the ice cream eaten in this study contained large amounts of sugar. On the positive side, however, the vitamin E and the oatmeal offered some protection against this dietary disaster.

Taking vitamin C and E supplements and choosing healthier foods offers the best protection against heart disease. However, these studies show that if you do indulge in high-fat/high-carbohydrate foods, it's smart to take vitamin E and vitamin C right before, or with your meal.

Vitamin E Might Help Reverse Clogged Arteries

There is evidence from animal and human studies that vitamin E may help *reverse* heart disease. Researchers have found that in monkeys, our close biological relatives, clogged arteries induced by a high-fat diet can not only be prevented, but can also be reversed by modest amounts of vitamin E. In a six-year research project, Anthony J. Verlangieri, Ph.D., of the University of Mississippi's Atherosclerosis Research Laboratory, fed monkeys a high-fat diet that caused their arteries to become clogged and blocked.

When the monkeys were also given vitamin E, the extent of arterial blockage dropped 60 to 80 percent. More remarkable was the fact that arteries that were seriously clogged began to open up.

Similarly, Howard N. Hodis, M.D., of the University of Southern California School of Medicine, Los Angeles, monitored the condition of people who had undergone bypass surgery. He found that patients who took 100–450 IU of vitamin E daily developed smaller lesions, or cholesterol deposits, on their arteries, than other bypass patients who didn't take vitamin E supplements. So, even if you've already had bypass surgery, vitamin E can help you. And, as we noted earlier in this chapter, a recent analysis of five large-scale, published trials led to the conclusion that many patients with pre-existing heart disease who took alpha-tocopherol supplements had a reduced risk of a nonfatal heart attack.

Vitamin E and Bypass Surgery

It's never too late to start taking vitamin E. But if you're scheduled for heart surgery, you should discuss taking vitamin E with your heart doctor. There is substantial research showing that vitamin E and other antioxidant vitamins can reduce the risk of complications, not only from bypass surgery, but also from balloon angioplasty and other types of surgical procedures.

During bypass surgery, blood flow is temporarily stopped so surgeons can graft new arteries. When the flow of oxygen-rich blood is replenished, large numbers of free radicals are generated, and these radicals can damage the heart. To protect against the free radical damage that's common with surgery, an increasing number of heart surgeons give their patients supplements of vitamin E and other antioxidants, such as vitamin C and coenzyme Q_{10}, before surgery. But a word of caution here. Due to its blood-thinning action, it is not advisable to take vitamin E before surgery if you're also taking a prescription blood-thinner like warfarin (Coumadin), without the guidance of a doctor knowledgeable about vitamin E.

Doctors' Opinions about Vitamin E

A growing number of doctors are warming up to the idea of taking vitamin E and are recommending supplements to their patients. Years ago, doctors had no explanation for why vitamin E could prevent and effectively treat heart disease. Today, most doctors understand that vitamin E is an antioxidant that protects against heart-damaging free radicals.

In general, Western medicine has long been skeptical of the health benefits of vitamin supplements. It has taken a long time for doctors to adjust to the idea that high doses of vitamins might be good for health. For example, it's difficult for many surgeons to recommend a nonsurgical way to treat heart disease. They have been trained as surgeons, and that's how they make their living.

Another problem has been physician education. In medical schools, doctors learn a lot about anatomy, physiology, diseases, and treatments, but almost nothing about nutrition. Dietitians are schooled in nutrition, but even they often underestimate the health benefits of vitamin supplements in amounts beyond the too-conservative RDAs. After medical school, much of a physician's ongoing education is strongly influenced by large drug companies. These companies are interested in selling expensive, proprietary drugs, not inexpensive vitamins. So drugs, not vitamins, are what physicians hear about most, particularly from the drug representatives who visit frequently and inundate them with drug samples and reams of copy on the special qualities of their product.

Nobel laureate Linus Pauling, Ph.D., once said, "If a doctor isn't 'up' on something, he's 'down' on it." If your doctor tells you vitamin E is a waste of money, he or she is either uninformed, irresponsible, or behind the times in his or her medical knowledge. In a typical year, medical journals publish about 500 scientific reports on vitamin E research.

Antioxidants
Substances, including vitamin E, that act like body-guards. They limit damage from free radicals by donating electrons to them.

If you decide to stick with this doctor, and to entrust your health to him, it's up to you to educate him—and to protect your health by taking vitamin E. Bring up the subject in a polite, non-threatening way. You could even share this book with him.

Even though your doctor may be skeptical about a "popular" (rather than medical) book, point him to the scientific references at the back of this book. He'll be able to use these references to look up everything he needs to know about vitamin E. If your doctor doesn't want to look up the references, and isn't willing to have a two-way conversation with you, the handwriting is on the wall: this doctor isn't a good one. Find another one.

How Much Vitamin E Is Needed to Benefit the Heart?

In general, 400 IU of natural vitamin E should be an ideal dose for most people to prevent coronary heart disease. The natural form of vitamin E is superior to the synthetic form, and we'll explain more about the difference in Chapter 8. If you have very serious heart disease, or are taking prescription drugs for your heart, tell your doctor of your interest in vitamin E. Sometimes people can reduce their intake of prescription drugs after they start taking vitamin E, but this is best done with a physician's guidance.

Even if you eat a healthy diet, you're probably not getting enough vitamin E. The amount most commonly recommended to benefit the heart—400 IU—is impossible to get from foods alone. You'd have to eat 1,000 almonds (or one pound of sunflower seeds)—8,000 calories worth of food—to obtain this amount of vitamin E.

CHAPTER 2

REDUCING THE
RISK OF CANCER

We tend to think of cancer as a single disease, but there are more than 100 kinds of cancer. They can cause different symptoms and be brought on by various factors, but virtually all develop because of damage by free radicals, the same hazardous molecules that also cause heart disease.

The good news is that there are many preventive measures we can take to reduce our risk for cancer. One of the most important is to take vitamin E. In this chapter, we'll look at how cancer develops, the relationship between vitamin E and cancer prevention, some of the ways vitamin E is thought to protect against specific types of cancer, and the forms of vitamin E that may be the most protective.

Vitamin E Reduces Cancer Risk

The scientific evidence shows that vitamin E can reduce cancer risk. According to an article in *Cancer Causes and Control,* researchers analyzed fifty-nine human studies on vitamin/mineral supplements and cancer risk and found that, of all the supplements studied, vitamin E supplements were the most strongly associated with a reduced cancer risk. Many studies have also found that high levels of vitamin E in the body are associated with a lower risk of cancer, whereas low levels are associated with a greater risk. These trends have been identified with breast cancer, cervical cancer and cervical dysplasia, colon cancer, lung cancer, and throat cancer.

Although vitamin E can reduce the risk of cancer, do not view it as a treatment (though it may be helpful in conjunction with other treatments). In some studies that have found no anticancer benefits from vitamin E, the participants have smoked for years or eaten a poor diet. Smoking and an unhealthy diet are strong risk factors for cancer, so vitamin E isn't a magic bullet that can totally erase the deleterious, cumulative effects brought on by years of unhealthy living. It is, however, an essential nutrient the body needs to function properly and help ward off diseases.

How Cancer Develops

Cancer is a disease in which normal cell growth goes awry. It usually (but not always) develops very slowly. Most cancers begin when free radicals damage the deoxyribonucleic acid (DNA, or genetic material) within your cells. Malignant tumors can result from the buildup of cells dividing uncontrollably, then they tend to spread and cause new malignant growths.

DNA is a set of biological instructions that tells your cells how to function normally. When DNA becomes damaged, the instructions that tell cells to perform properly become garbled. Even when a cell becomes cancerous, the immune system can often destroy it before it replicates and becomes established as a cancer. But when free radical damage occurs in enough of your cells, cancerous cells can overwhelm the beleaguered immune system and can proliferate, accumulate and spread.

Free radicals are byproducts of normal cellular processes, so they're a natural part of living. But free radicals also are generated by exposure to pollutants, radiation and chemicals. Modern living, therefore, often tips the balance between free radicals and antioxidants (free radical quenchers) toward too many free radicals.

Tobacco smoke increases free radicals significantly, which is why smokers have a very high risk of most cancers (not just lung cancer). Because a big part of the process that leads to cancer involves damage from too many free radicals, the best way to protect your body against cancer is to supplement your diet with such antioxidants as vitamin E, and to avoid the unnecessary free radical production that such behavior as smoking causes.

How Vitamin E Protects against Cancer

Vitamin E protects against cancer in several ways. First and foremost, as a component of cell membranes, vitamin E helps prevent these membranes from becoming damaged by free radicals from a wide variety of sources, including chemicals, radiation, and toxins.

Vitamin E also can prevent nitrites (compounds found in smoked, cured and pickled foods) from forming nitrosamines, which are strong tumor promoters. It may also assist or accelerate the body's metabolism of carcinogenic, or cancer-causing, substances. In other words, vitamin E may help the body get rid of potential cancer-causing agents in the body more quickly.

In addition, vitamin E appears to block the formation of blood vessels in tumors. This is significant because tumors need their own network of blood vessels for nourishment in order to grow.

Creating these blood vessels is a process called angiogenesis. According to cell and rodent studies, vitamin E has anti-angiogenic properties.

Angiogenesis
Describes the formation of blood vessels, which tumors need to receive nourishment and grow.

This anti-angiogenic property is particularly true of the "succinate" form (d-alpha-tocopheryl succinate) of vitamin E. In addition, there is growing evidence that vitamin E plays a role in normal gene expression, or activation. It's very possible that vitamin E maintains normal gene activity and helps turn off the abnormal gene activity characteristic of tumors.

Other research shows that cancerous tumors generate large numbers of their own free radicals, thereby creating endless mutations to circumvent various types of chemotherapeutic drugs. These drugs can be target-specific, so mutated forms of cancer cells may escape the drugs' cancer-fighting effects, allowing the cancer to thrive. By quenching free radicals, vitamin E may slow down the mutation rate in cancer, enabling other treatments to fight it.

Probably the most important way vitamin E helps ward off cancer is by boosting the immune system. As mentioned earlier, cancerous cells can develop—many experts think all people have some cancer cells in their bodies—but cancerous tumors won't take hold as long as our immune systems are strong and primed to scavenge those cells.

Vitamin E supplementation has been shown to boost the immune system in a variety of ways, including increasing the activity of natural killer (NK) cells. NK cells are "Rambo"-type cells, which can recognize cells that have gone bad; they're fully armed and ready to kill cancerous cells on the spot before the cells can divide and cause harm.

This means that supplemental vitamin E helps keep your immune cells in a vigorous state, ready to attack the first cancer cells they find.

Though Not a Cure, Vitamin E Can Inhibit Cancer Cell Growth

At this time, there's no research to indicate that vitamin E can reverse cancer in humans (in other words, do not try to use vitamin E as a "cure" for cancer). There is, however, one particular type of vitamin E, d-alpha-tocopheryl succinate, which has been found to inhibit the growth of cancer cells in cell cultures (dishes of cells in a laboratory) and rodent experiments. And there is another group of vitamin E molecules, called tocotrienols, which has also been found to kill human breast cancer cells grown in cell cultures. So far, the research is preliminary, but scientists are excited about the promise of both forms of vitamin E against cancer.

Although one day certain types of vitamin E and other nutrients may be used routinely against existing cancer, the best approach is to begin taking vitamin E now to help prevent cancer. Prevention is always the best policy, especially for cancer, which can be a devastating, deadly, and emotionally wrenching disease. To put all this a slightly different way: If either of us were diagnosed with cancer, we would take supplements of the d-alpha-tocopheryl succinate form of vitamin E in addition to pursuing other types of therapies. We would not rely on vitamin E alone, and neither should you.

Vitamin E Reduces the Risk of Prostate Cancer

Vitamin E supplementation significantly lowers

the risk of prostate cancer, according to recent findings reported in the *Journal of the National Cancer Institute*. In the study, Ollie P. Heinonen, M.D., D.Sc., and his colleagues at the University of Helsinki tracked the health of 29,000 men for six years. The men taking vitamin E were found to be 32 percent less likely to develop prostate cancer and 41 percent less likely to die from the disease if they did develop it. And these beneficial effects were seen within two years of starting the supplementation.

The results of this study are especially significant because the men were smokers at above-average risk of cancer. The researchers acknowledged that the simple intervention of taking a vitamin E supplement might help prevent prostate cancer, the most frequently diagnosed cancer in men, but even they were surprised by how strong the benefits were. This study used a relatively low dose—50 IU—of vitamin E, but a higher dose—400 IU—has greater overall benefits to the heart and, likely, to the prostate.

Prostate Gland

The doughnut-shaped gland below the bladder in men, which secretes a solution that aids in sperm movement and health.

Cell studies point to a role for vitamin E in prostate cancer protection, too. In a recent study published in the journal *Nutrition and Cancer* in 2000, natural vitamin-E succinate (d-alpha-tocopheryl succinate) stopped the growth of two types of prostate cancer cells and actually caused these cells to self-destruct. Vitamin E didn't hurt normal prostate cells, though.

Vitamin E May Offer Protection against Breast Cancer

Vitamin E may protect against breast cancer as

well. Research with animals suggests that vitamin E can compensate somewhat for a genetic defect that increases the risk of breast cancer. Some people have a genetic defect that results in low production of catalase, an antioxidant enzyme the body produces. Without sufficient catalase, cells have trouble neutralizing the free radicals that can cause breast cancer.

Japanese researchers at the Okayama University Medical School studied mice that did not produce enough catalase. They found that catalase-deficient mice were more likely than normal mice to develop breast cancer. But when the researchers added vitamin E to the mice's diet, the mice were far less likely to develop breast cancer.

Could vitamin E benefit people in the same way? According to the researchers, who published their findings in the *Japanese Journal of Cancer Research*, "vitamin E intrinsically has a protective effect against the development of mammary tumor, and this may apply . . . to humans." Most of us don't know whether we're producing insufficient catalase or not. However, this research suggests that taking vitamin E over a lifetime may reduce the risk of breast cancer in those individuals who unknowingly produce low amounts of catalase.

Vitamin E Protects the Skin

Vitamin E protects the skin from free radical damage, too. The skin is regularly exposed to ultraviolet (UV) radiation from sunlight that generates large numbers of free radicals, which age the skin and greatly increase the risk of skin cancer. Skin cancer is of great concern because it is the most prevalent type of cancer, and its incidence among Americans is steadily increasing.

Research in rodents has found that both internal and external use of vitamin E protects the skin from the initial damage that can occur from excessive exposure to UV radiation. It also raises the levels of protective antioxidants in the skin and reduces suppression of the immune system, which often occurs as a result of too much exposure to sunlight. Via these mechanisms, it makes the body better able to protect itself against skin cancer.

Vitamin E Protects against Mouth, Throat, and Colorectal Cancer

What's more, vitamin E helps protect against precancerous growths in the mouth and throat. These growths are predominantly found in people who smoke tobacco or drink excessive amounts of alcohol—activities that generate large numbers of free radicals. In a study conducted by Steven Benner, M.D., of the University of Texas Anderson Cancer Center, Houston, patients with these growths were given 400 IU of vitamin E twice daily for twenty-four weeks. About a quarter of the patients had a greater than 50 percent decrease in the size of their precancerous lesions and another quarter had a complete disappearance of the growths.

Another study—this one with 29,000 male cigarette smokers—found that 50 IU per day of vitamin E for five to eight years led to a slightly reduced risk of developing colorectal cancer. Larger doses might have decreased their risk of disease even more. Smokers taking beta-carotene or a placebo didn't experience this protective effect. These are some good examples of how vitamin E can quench free radicals from a variety of sources and thus protect against many different forms of cancer.

Supplementing with Vitamin E for Cancer Protection

Vitamin E is recognized as the key antioxidant for protecting cellular membranes (walls) against free radical damage, so your health will certainly benefit from taking vitamin E. As with coronary heart disease, 400 IU of natural vitamin E seems to be an effective and safe dose. But research indicates that a diverse selection of antioxidants may be more important for protecting the body against free radical damage than high doses of a single antioxidant.

Antioxidants other than vitamin E include vitamin C, alpha-lipoic acid, beta-carotene and other carotenoids (such as lutein and lycopene), co-enzyme Q_{10}, selenium, and zinc. Different antioxidants scavenge different types of free radicals, so a combination of antioxidants forms a stronger antioxidant shield to protect the body against cancer and other degenerative diseases.

Antioxidants also work synergistically with each other. Vitamin C, for example, recycles vitamin E that has been used up; selenium works in concert with vitamin E; and zinc is needed to maintain normal blood concentrations of vitamin E. Taking a combination of antioxidants, therefore, better ensures that you'll get the most mileage out of the vitamin E you take.

CHAPTER 3

BOOSTING IMMUNITY AND QUENCHING INFLAMMATION

Vitamin E's ability to protect against heart disease and cancer has been the focus of much research. However, its ability to boost the immune system has gone largely unnoticed until recent years. Your immune system bolsters your defenses against colds and other infections. This chapter will cover the ways in which vitamin E enhances immunity and helps protect you against everyday minor illnesses and more serious infections, while also providing safe anti-inflammatory benefits.

Vitamin E Enhances Immunity

Several studies show that vitamin E boosts the immune system and can enhance resistance to infection. This is particularly important for older people, because the immune system declines with age and this leads to an increased susceptibility to illness.

In one study, Simin N. Meydani, D.V.M., Ph.D., of Tufts University, gave vitamin E to a group of men and women sixty-five years of age and older. Subjects taking 200 IU each day for about four months showed significant improvements on various tests that assess the immune system's ability to ward off diseases. The subjects' immune responses actually behaved more like those of forty-year-olds than sixty-five- or seventy-year-olds.

Furthermore, the incidence of self-reported illnesses, such as colds, declined by about 30 percent.

In other studies, vitamin E has been found to boost the immune responses of young people. Therefore, vitamin E might keep you from being sick as often, though the effect will likely be subtle and long term instead of quick and dramatic.

The Health Consequences of Vitamin E Deficiency

A deficiency of vitamin E can make you not only more susceptible to illness, but also more prone to virus mutations that can lead to serious disease. It's well known that nutritional deficiencies reduce the ability of the immune system to fight infections.

T Cells
Immune cells that fight off foreign invaders in the body, including bacteria, cancer cells, viruses, and more.

Vitamin E deficiencies are associated with decreased immune function and decreased differentiation of immature T cells, which fight off foreign invaders like bacteria, cancer cells, viruses, and others. Basically, deficiencies of vitamin E prevent your immune system from mounting an effective counterattack against bacteria and viruses. But there has been a recent, significant twist in this field.

In groundbreaking studies, Melinda Beck, Ph.D., of the University of North Carolina at Chapel Hill, and Orville Levander, Ph.D., of the U.S. Department of Agriculture, discovered that deficiencies of vitamin E or the mineral selenium in a person or animal could turn a common virus into a deadly, rapidly producing strain.

Beck and Levander studied the Coxsackie virus, which infects about 20 million Americans annually and usually causes no more than coldlike symptoms, diarrhea, or a sore throat. However, when a person or animal is deficient in vitamin E or selenium (a mineral that works in tandem with vitamin E), the virus can mutate into a strain that inflames the heart muscle, leading to cardiomyopathy and heart failure.

Adequate levels of both nutrients, though, prevent mutations of the virus. This research provides one more convincing reason to take supplemental vitamin E, as well as selenium. But there may be more reasons in the future: Beck and Levander are currently looking into how deficiencies of vitamin E and selenium might cause other viruses, such as cold and flu viruses, to mutate.

How Vitamin E Improves Immunity

The immune system mounts an amazingly complex defense against invaders, and vitamin E stimulates many parts of this defense. Specifically, vitamin E has been found to:

- improve the function of phagocytes (cells that act as biological "Pac-Men" against a broad range of microorganisms);

- stimulate activity of natural killer cells (which destroy cancer and virus-infected cells);

- enhance the body's ability to produce antibodies (which tag or damage viruses); and

- lower levels of prostaglandin E2, an inflammation-causing substance.

Through all these mechanisms, vitamin E acts as a powerful, broad-spectrum, immune enhancer. And, in addition to stimulating immunity, vitamin E protects the immune system from the wear and tear of constantly defending the body from unwanted invaders. Although it's surprising to many people, immune cells like phagocytes generate enormous quantities of free radicals to kill bacteria, yet these immune cells are highly susceptible to damage from free radicals themselves. Vitamin E, of course, quenches free radicals, protecting healthy cells—including immune cells—from damage.

If you're wondering about the best dose for boosting your immunity, that depends on your state of health. Doses of 200–400 IU of vitamin E daily are beneficial for most people. Higher doses of vitamin E (as well as other nutrients) may be beneficial for those with severe immunity problems.

Vitamin E's Benefits for Those with AIDS

Vitamin E can help those infected with AIDS (acquired immune deficiency syndrome). Here's why: Free radicals are known to promote the replication of the HIV virus, which causes AIDS. In animal studies, vitamin E has been shown to indirectly inhibit replication of the HIV virus by quenching free radicals and by stimulating various parts of the immune system.

A number of studies have found that people infected with HIV have low levels of vitamin E and other nutrients in addition to high amounts of free radicals. One recent study, conducted in Toronto, found that supplements of vitamins E and C reduced virus levels in people infected with HIV. All of this research suggests that vitamin E may be beneficial for treating HIV infection, but more studies in humans are needed to confirm this.

It's important to recognize that people with

HIV and AIDS may need far more than the standard, low RDA levels of vitamins. There are many reasons for this, not the least being that many patients with AIDS suffer from diarrhea, which promotes nutrient loss. Researchers have found that patients with HIV and AIDS have low blood levels of most vitamins and minerals, and that very high supplemental amounts are usually needed to achieve normal blood levels of these nutrients.

Does Vitamin E Exacerbate Autoimmune Diseases?

Since vitamin E boosts immunity, it's only natural to wonder whether vitamin E might exacerbate auto-immune diseases—conditions in which the immune system interprets the body's normal cells as invaders and attacks them. There are theories about what makes the immune system attack the body's own cells, but much about autoimmunity remains a mystery.

Autoimmune Disease
A condition in which the immune system attacks the body's own cells, as if they were foreign invaders.

The simple answer is that vitamin E is not likely to overstimulate the immune system and aggravate autoimmune diseases. Autoimmune dis-eases always involve inflammation in the body. Vitamin E enhances certain types of immune cells and dampens others that are involved in inflammation. Anytime you have inflammation in the body, in fact, large numbers of free radicals accompany the inflammation, and vitamin E can serve as an antidote against these damaging molecules.

Vitamin E Helps in Lupus and Rheumatoid Arthritis

Vitamin E actually improves the symptoms of individuals with autoimmune conditions like lupus or rheumatoid arthritis, as long as it is taken in high enough doses. For example, in one study, people with lupus receiving 900–1,600 IU of vitamin E per day showed complete or almost complete clearing of symptoms. Lower dosages of 300 IU, however, had no effect. People with rheumatoid arthritis, another chronic inflammatory disease, have also benefited from supplementation, experiencing a lessening of pain and stiffness, with doses ranging from 400–1,200 IU per day.

Vitamin E seems to work well in conjunction with standard arthritis treatments, too. One example is a recent study in which thirty patients with rheumatoid disease were given either a standard drug-treatment regimen, a standard drug treatment plus a combination of low-potency antioxidants, or a high dose of vitamin E (400 IU three times a day) in combination with standard drug treatment.

Patients who took the antioxidant combination or vitamin E with the standard treatment had better control of arthritis symptoms from the first month of treatment than those who received only standard treatment. Patients who took vitamin E also had more significant improvements in disease severity, inflammation, and morning stiffness than those taking only standard drug treatment.

Vitamin E Counters Inflammation

As an antioxidant, vitamin E does a lot to counter inflammation, which is not only involved in autoimmune diseases, but also in injuries. We've already described the damage that free radicals can cause to genes, fats, proteins and more. As if that weren't devastating enough to the body, free radicals also stimulate and intensify inflammation.

They do this by turning on genes that promote inflammation.

As an antioxidant, vitamin E can quench free radicals before they have a chance to induce inflammation. This powerful vitamin also reduces important promoters of inflammation, including C-reactive protein (CRP), adhesion molecules (which help white blood cells adhere to normal cells), and interleukin-6 (IL-6). C-reactive protein is such an important marker of impending health problems that it requires a bit more explanation.

C-Reactive Protein Indicates Inflammation

CRP is a key marker of inflammation throughout the body, and high levels have been linked to a dramatically increased risk of heart attack, physical trauma, and serious infections.

High cholesterol and high homocysteine levels are associated with increased heart disease and heart-attack risk, and many people worry about these risk factors. But high levels of CRP are now considered even more predictive of a heart attack. CRP is found in atherosclerotic lesions and is related to the lesion's rupture, which can lead to blood vessel clots and, in turn, to blood-flow blockage and heart attacks.

Other conditions linked to high CRP levels are blood-sugar problems, including diabetes, insulin resistance, and Syndrome X (which you'll learn about in Chapter 6). Overweight people and smok - ers, as well as those with Alzheimer's disease, arthritis, and cancer, tend to have higher-than-normal CRP levels, too. Some of the latest research suggests that supplementing with vitamin E can lower CRP a great deal. If you wish, you can ask your physician to measure your CRP levels.

How Vitamin E Quells Inflammation

Vitamin E's benefit in preventing LDL cholesterol from being oxidized is important in how it helps quell inflammation. As we described more generally in the first chapter, white blood cells go after oxidized LDL in the inflammation process, using an arsenal of free radicals themselves as poison to destroy the oxidized LDL.

But free radicals that leak out of the white blood cells cause more inflammation and can even penetrate artery walls where they gobble up more LDL, stick there, and grow into lesions. Smooth muscle cells try to block off the problem area by covering it, but this leads to even worse blockage. And there's more bad news: sometimes part of a lesion will break off, leading to a potentially dangerous clot that blocks the flow of blood.

But preventing LDL from being oxidized can keep the process described above from happening. Vitamin E, as you've learned, also keeps inflammation under control by inhibiting a variety of other pro-inflammatory substances, including CRP and IL-6.

Vitamin E supplementation appears to be the best natural method of lowering CRP levels. In one study, the effects of various antioxidants on fifty-seven people with type II diabetes were investigated. As reported in *Diabetes Care*, 800 IU of natural vitamin E daily for four weeks cut CRP levels by 50 percent. Neither 500 mg of vitamin C daily nor tomato juice (rich in lycopene) daily for four weeks could match this result.

In another study, people with diabetes, healthy people, and women with heart disease took 1,200 IU of natural vitamin E daily for three months. All of these groups averaged 30 percent drops in CRP, and their levels of interleukin-6 fell by 50 percent.

Vitamin E, therefore, not only acts as an immune booster but also as an anti-inflammatory agent. Through these two mechanisms, it can protect us from minor illnesses and chronic diseases.

CHAPTER 4

PRESERVING
THE MIND

Vitamin E is critical for proper brain and nerve function, and supplements of it have been found to have beneficial effects against such brain and nervous system disorders as Alzheimer's disease, Parkinson's disease, and tardive dyskinesia. This chapter will cover the important roles of vitamin E in brain and nerve health and how vitamin E is believed to protect against these devastating diseases.

Vitamin E Is Important for Brain Health

The brain contains large amounts of polyunsaturated fatty acids (PUFAs), the types of fats most prone to free radical damage. When the fatty acids in one brain cell become damaged, they can trigger a chain reaction in which many fatty acids throughout the brain become damaged.

Vitamin E, though, can halt this wildfire reaction before it begins: it's the most important fat-soluble antioxidant to shield fatty tissues, like those in the brain, from damage. Taking supplemental vitamin E, therefore, helps promote optimal brain health and should lower the risk of Alzheimer's and other degenerative diseases associated with free radical damage.

Vitamin E Can Slow the Progression of Alzheimer's Disease

Vitamin E isn't a cure for Alzheimer's disease, but it can slow the progression of this disease more than a leading drug used for this purpose. In a recent study reported in *The New England Journal of Medicine,* Mary Sano, Ph.D., of Columbia University's College of Physicians and Surgeons, New York, and her colleagues gave patients with severe Alzheimer's disease a large dose of either vitamin E (2,000 IU), selegiline (a drug used to treat Parkinson's disease), a combination of the two, or a placebo daily for two years.

Vitamin E delayed the progression of end-stage Alzheimer's by almost eight months compared with the placebo, or slightly longer than with the selegiline. Patients who took vitamin E showed 25 percent less decline in their ability to perform daily tasks like cooking, dressing, and eating. These kinds of abilities keep those with Alzheimer's at home rather than in a nursing facility and improve the quality of life for them. For a disease that has no known cure, these results are impressive.

> **Alzheimer's Disease**
> A degenerative brain disease caused by neuron dysfunction and death that causes problems with behavior, feelings, memory, and thinking.

Right after this study was published, the American Psychiatric Association gave its seal of approval to vitamin E, recommending it as a normal and appropriate part of the treatment for Alz - heimer's. Both the American Academy of Neurology and the Alzheimer's Association have also approved the recommendation of 1,000 IU of vitamin E twice daily to slow the progression of Alzheimer's. Another study is under way to see if vitamin E will be even more effective for those with early-stage Alzheimer's disease.

The authors of a placebo-controlled, clinical trial conducted by the Alzheimer's Disease Cooperative Study, published in the *American Journal of Clinical Nutrition,* concluded that vitamin E "may slow functional deterioration leading to nursing home placement." In the study, patients with moderately advanced Alzheimer's disease were treated with 2000 IU of vitamin E per day. The results of additional trials should help determine whether vitamin E can delay or prevent Alzheimer's disease in older people with mild cognitive problems.

How Vitamin E Helps in Alzheimer's Disease

Here's why vitamin E may slow Alzheimer's disease and possibly even prevent or delay its onset. Vitamin E seems to prevent oxidative damage from beta-amyloid, a substance found in high amounts in the brains of Alzheimer's disease patients. Vitamin E maintains cell-membrane flexibility, and brain cells that have flexible membranes function more efficiently.

Cell membranes act like the walls and doors of cells. As long as they are flexible, they allow other important nutrients into cells and waste products out. If the membranes of brain cells start to get rigid, important nutrients can't get in and cellular waste products just keep accumulating inside these brain cells, causing poor function and, eventually, their destruction which can lead to Alzheimer's disease.

Supplementing with Vitamin E for Protection of Brain Health

You should take vitamin E to protect your overall health, and doing this should reduce your risk of developing Alzheimer's disease over the long term. It's likely that the longer you take vitamin E, the more protected you will be against Alzheimer's disease. Although some Alzheimer's studies have used 2,000 IU of vitamin E daily, much less is probably needed for long-term prevention. Again, an ideal preventive dose would seem to be about 400 IU daily.

Beta-amyloid is the abnormal protein that accumulates in the brains of Alzheimer's patients. In lab and rodent experiments, researchers have found that nerve cells die when they are exposed to beta-amyloid. But when vitamin E is added, the cells stay healthy. Many researchers in the field believe vitamin E can act preventively against Alzheimer's disease and they take vitamin E for this reason.

If you're young, taking steps to prevent Alzheimer's disease may be the furthest thing from your mind. It shouldn't be, though. Alzheimer's disease is the fourth leading cause of death in the United States. More than 4 million older Americans have the disease, and that number is expected to skyrocket as more of us live into our eighties and nineties.

Vitamin E's Effects on Other Brain and Nerve Conditions

Tardive dyskinesia is another condition that vitamin E might help. This is a condition characterized by involuntary muscle movements. It often affects long-term alcoholics and people who have been treated with antipsychotic drugs.

Like Alzheimer's disease, tardive dyskinesia is believed to be caused by free radical damage. Several studies have found vitamin E effective in treating tardive dyskinesia, especially in those who have had the disease for five years or less. In one scientifically controlled study of twenty-eight patients, a daily intake of 1,600 IU of vitamin E for two to three months was found to reduce involuntary muscle movements by one-third.

Parkinson's disease involves progressive degeneration of nerve cells in the brain. Symptoms include incapacitating tremors, rigidity and loss of balance. There's some conflicting evidence on the effectiveness of vitamin E against Parkinson's, perhaps because several studies used synthetic vitamin E, which is not well assimilated. However, vitamin E still appears to be helpful. In a large-scale study of 5,342 people in the Netherlands, researchers found the risk of Parkinson's disease went up as the consumption of vitamin E went down.

Parkinson's Disease
A disease that involves progressive degeneration of nerve cells in the brain and causes loss of balance, rigidity, and tremors.

Since free radicals are believed to be at work in Parkinson's disease, researchers at the Columbia University Department of Neurology gave high doses of vitamin E (3,200 IU), coupled with 3 grams of vitamin C, to Parkinson's patients. The researchers found that those on the antioxidant therapy went 2.5 years longer before requiring drug therapy to treat their symptoms than those who received no antioxidants. The doctors conducting this trial concluded that, "the progression of Parkinson's disease may be slowed by administration of these antioxidants."

Can Vitamin E Improve Memory?

There's no direct evidence to prove that vitamin E enhances memory, but it does promote healthy brain function and healthy brain function is needed for normal memory recall. If vitamin E is taken regularly, it's logical to think that it might help memory slightly. Researchers recently found a correlation between the amount of vitamin E per unit of blood cholesterol and memory perform-ance among a multiethnic sample of 4,809 older people, based on data from the Third National Health and Nutrition Examination Survey.

In addition, brain function naturally declines as we age, but vitamin E can slow this aging process. In an experiment involving mice, supplemental vi-tamin E (in amounts equivalent to a human dose of 400 IU per day) was found to prolong the life of brain cells by preventing or delaying free radical damage to a crucial strand of proteins called band-3 proteins. This research suggests that the cells which perform thinking and memory func-tions are among those that receive the most pro-tection from vitamin E supplementation.

Taking vitamin E is a good, long-term strategy to support brain health and keep you mentally sharp. If your memory has faltered some and you're actively trying to improve it, though, try taking acetyl-L-carnitine and phosphatidyl serine (other nutrients which appear to be significant memory-enhancers) in addition to vitamin E.

CHAPTER 5

IMPROVING SEXUAL HEALTH

In the 1920s, researchers discovered that vitamin E was necessary for reproduction in rats and people started referring to vitamin E as the sex vitamin. Although vitamin E isn't an aphrodisiac, it turns out that it does help a wide variety of conditions related to the reproductive system—everything from impotence and infertility in men to menopausal hot flashes, premenstrual syndrome, and sore breasts in women. In this chapter, we'll sort through the truths and misconceptions about vitamin E as a sex vitamin.

Vitamin E May Help Impotence

Impotence, called erectile dysfunction in the medical field, affects millions of men worldwide. In one study, 52 percent of male subjects forty- to seventy-years-old were affected. Vitamin E can help some men with erectile dysfunction, but not in the same way as the prescription drug Viagra. Viagra can improve sexual performance immediately, but it can also be dangerous and should be avoided by those with heart or eye disease. Vitamin E works in a more subtle way to improve sexual performance and, of course, heart health.

Many factors, including aging, alcohol consumption, chronic illness, diabetes, high blood pressure, medication, and smoking, can have a negative effect on the ability to have erections. However, many cases of impotence are actually related to cardiovascular disease. Basically, the blood vessels of the penis can become damaged and narrowed from a buildup of arterial plaque just like the blood vessels that surround the heart. So anything that improves cardiovascular disease —such as vitamin E—may help impotency. Vitamin E also improves circulation or blood flow to all tissues, including those in the penis. Every condition improves with better blood flow.

Some scientists think that changes in protein kinase C and free radical production in diabetes could be part of the cause of erectile dysfunction among diabetic men. In an animal-cell study, vitamin E (the alpha-tocopherol form) reduced free radical production and protein kinase C in smooth muscle cells from the penis. Future human studies should shed light on the potential of vitamin E to help men with erectile dysfunction.

Vitamin E's Effects on Improving Fertility

Vitamin E shows promise in improving fertility as well. Several studies, published in *Fertility and Sterility*, have reported that infertile men have low levels of antioxidants in their semen and high levels of free radicals, which can deform sperm and prevent fertilization of the egg.

Vitamin E strengthens and protects the cell membranes of sperm and apparently helps them go that extra inch to father a child. In one study, Ami Amit, M.D., of Israel, gave men with normal sperm counts but low fertilization rates 200 IU of vitamin E daily for three months. The vitamin E lowered free radical levels in the men's semen and boosted their fertilization rate by 30 percent.

It takes at least three months for vitamins to have an effect in fertility, mainly because it takes that long for sperm to mature. Infertile couples should supplement with both vitamin E and a high-potency multivitamin for several months before trying to conceive. If you smoke, try to stop because tobacco smoke inflicts free radical damage on sperm.

Natural Vitamin E—Important for a Healthy Pregnancy

Vitamin E not only seems to help women conceive, it also is important for a healthy pregnancy. You can and should take vitamin E while pregnant for the health of you and your baby. Vitamin E can help protect against complications that sometimes occur during pregnancy and against those that can occur in babies who are born prematurely. It's important, though, to ask your doctor for prenatal supplements that contain natural vitamin E instead of synthetic.

Synthetic vitamin E is the type found in most prenatal supplements, but a recent study reported in the *American Journal of Clinical Nutrition* found that the human placenta can deliver natural vitamin E to the fetus 3.5 times more efficiently than it can the synthetic supplement. Pregnancy is the most important time in life to ensure optimal nutrition. Give you and your baby the best by asking your doctor specifically for a prenatal supplement that contains natural vitamin E.

Vitamin E Can Ease Fibrocystic Breast Pain and PMS

Vitamin E is important for protecting the health of women who aren't pregnant, too. First, vitamin E offers relief in fibrocystic breast disease, which is not really a disease but a group of benign conditions affecting the breast. The condition, which is very common in premenopausal women, usually involves cysts, lumps, pain, or tenderness in the breasts.

Several studies show that, for many women with fibrocystic breast disease symptoms, vitamin E appears to be quite effective in relieving the condition. In one study of twenty-six women with fibrocystic breast disease, 85 percent (twenty-two women) of those who received 600 IU of vitamin E daily for eight weeks responded to treatment.

In a study of twelve women taking vitamin E, benign cysts decreased in number and size and, in ten of the women, there was a total disappearance of breast tenderness and cysts. In addition to taking vitamin E, an important strategy for alleviating symptoms of fibrocystic breast disease is to strictly avoid caffeine (found in coffee, tea, cola and chocolate). This alone can totally eradicate the symptoms of this disease in many women.

Fibrocystic Breasts

Describes a group of benign conditions of the breast, including cysts, lumps, pain and tenderness.

Vitamin E appears to work well for some women with premenstrual syndrome (PMS), but not for everyone. Most of the research on vitamin E and PMS has focused primarily on breast tenderness, but at least one study suggests vitamin E may help lessen other PMS symptoms including depression, fatigue, headache, insomnia, and nervous tension.

Whether or not vitamin E by itself relieves premenstrual tension, you should take supplemental vitamin E as good preventive medicine to protect yourself against heart disease, the leading killer of women. The best strategy to overcome PMS is a comprehensive one: Take vitamin E, but try adding supplements of B-complex vitamins, chromium, magnesium, and zinc, which have proven to be of value for some women. And try avoiding all forms of sugar in your diet, as this is also effective for alleviating PMS symptoms in many women.

Vitamin E Can Reduce Hot Flashes

Finally, vitamin E offers relief for menopausal women who experience hot flashes and other uncomfortable symptoms. Most of the research regarding vitamin E for hot flashes was actually conducted in the 1940s. Several studies found vitamin E effective in relieving hot flashes (as well as menopausal vaginal complaints) when compared with a dummy pill. Since then, many health-minded women have used vitamin E for these purposes, though no follow-up tests had been done.

Recently, however, researchers at the Mayo Clinic found that women can experience a reduction of hot flashes in as little as a month of supplementing with 800 IU of vitamin E. The study was interesting because it involved 120 breast cancer survivors who couldn't take estrogen replacement therapy (ERT). Although ERT is the most common treatment for such menopausal symptoms as hot flashes, breast cancer survivors can't use it because it often stimulates the growth of breast cancer cells.

The breast cancer survivors who took vitamin E experienced a small but statistically significant decrease in hot-flash activity after just four weeks, with no risk of side effects. Taking vitamin E for longer periods of time probably would provide even more beneficial effects.

For women who cannot use estrogen replacement therapy—or for those who simply prefer not to—vitamin E appears to be a mild, natural substitute to ease hot flashes. It doesn't, however, address all menopausal health concerns, so work with a nutritionally minded health professional to devise a complete nutrition strategy if you experience difficulties during and after menopause.

(CHAPTER 6)

SLOWING THE AGING PROCESS AND MORE

Throughout this book, you've read about vitamin E's ability to prevent free radical damage and protect against everything from heart disease to Alzheimer's disease. This chapter will cover a wide assortment of other health benefits from vitamin E—including its ability to slow the aging process, reduce the risk of cataracts, lessen exercise-induced fatigue, help heal burns and possibly even protect against wrinkles.

Vitamin E Slows Down the Aging Process

Vitamin E is one of a number of nutrients that seem to slow the aging process. The basic idea is that free radicals damage cells and, in effect, age them. As an antioxidant, vitamin E slows down this damage, as do other antioxidants like vitamin C and coenzyme Q_{10}. Your body is essentially composed of around 100 billion cells, and it stands to reason that slowing the aging of these individual cells will slow the aging of your entire body.

Another way to look at this is in terms of reducing your risk for some of the top age-related disease killers such as heart disease, cancer, and Alzheimer's disease. Scientific studies have shown pretty clearly that vitamin E reduces the risk of developing these diseases. It might not completely eliminate the risk—but for the sake of discussion, let's assume that vitamin E only delays the onset of these diseases. This means you might not develop heart disease until you're eighty years old, instead of sixty. If vitamin E delays the onset of these serious diseases by ten, twenty, or thirty years, you're going to live longer and more healthfully.

Realistically, then, vitamin E can slow the aging process—that is, the speed at which your body's cells age. It is not an "antiaging" vitamin in the technical sense, because aging is an inevitable process. Vitamin E will not turn a forty-year-old man into a teenager. However, it may help restore the heart function of a seventy-year-old to that of someone ten or twenty years younger. But remember that eating a good diet, exercising, and minimizing stresses in your life also retards the aging process.

Vitamin E Protects against Cataracts

Cataracts are an age-related condition that vitamin E can help you avoid. Vitamin E has been found to significantly reduce the risk of cataracts, which accounts for 42 percent of all vision loss and is the leading cause of blindness worldwide.

Cataract
Clouding of the normally transparent eye lens, impairing vision; often asso-ciated with aging and diabetes.

Free radicals from pollution and ultraviolet radiation damage the proteins that form the lens of the eye and cause cataracts, so it isn't surprising that vitamin E can delay the onset and slow the progression of cataracts. In a recent study, 744 older people who took vitamin E supplements lowered their risk of developing cataracts by 57 percent.

Vitamin E appears to benefit people with cortical cataracts (an opacity, or cloudy area, toward the outside of the eye lens) more than those with nuclear cataracts (an opacity in the center of the lens). In an eye-opening study, Simmi Kharb, Ph.D., of the Postgraduate Institute of Medical Sciences in Rohtak, India, found that patients with cortical cataracts had an almost 40 percent decrease in lens opacity after taking vitamin E supplements twice daily for a month. Patients with nuclear cataracts had a decrease of only 14 percent.

Similarly, vitamin E benefited cortical lens tissue more significantly in other ways—decreased free radical activity, increased antioxidant production, and increased vitamin E levels—than it benefited nuclear lens tissue. Even so, vitamin E did improve both kinds of cataracts among those studied, just to different degrees.

Vitamin E Is Helpful for Diabetics and Those with Syndrome X

Vitamin E also helps protect against two increasingly common diseases of aging—type II diabetes and Syndrome X. Type II diabetes is characterized by high blood sugar (glucose) levels and numerous symptoms, including fatigue, frequent thirst, frequent urination, and poor concentration. Syndrome X is the combination of abdominal obesity, elevated blood cholesterol or triglycerides, and high blood pressure.

Both diseases involve insulin resistance—a condition in which the glucose-lowering hormone insulin does not work efficiently—and high insulin levels at their core. Both conditions also accel-erate aging and carry a greatly increased risk of diseases associated with aging, including cardiovascular disease, mental deterioration, and some types of cancer.

Part of the disease process in type II diabetes is the result of free radicals spinning off from high glucose levels. Blood glucose increases free radical damage to cells, interferes with normal cell replication and actually kills cells. Anything you can do to reduce free radicals can hold off this health-damaging process. That's what vitamin E does.

By quenching free radicals, vitamin E also limits the formation of advanced glycation endproducts—AGEs, for short. AGEs quite literally age cells. One AGE that's found in the blood is called glycated hemoglobin. This is the standard marker that people with diabetes measure to see that their condition is being controlled. High levels of glycated hemoglobin signify high glucose levels. Vitamin E can help those with diabetes manage their glucose levels and can therefore reduce the formation of AGEs that lead to many diabetic complications.

Vitamin E can also lower glucose levels and help insulin work more normally, both in people with insulin resistance and in healthy people. In a recent Italian study, a regimen of 600 IU of vitamin E daily for two weeks lowered glucose levels and free radical formation among diabetic subjects. In a study conducted by Giuseppe Paolisso, M.D., of the University of Naples, Italy, vitamin E improved glucose tolerance and insulin action in healthy people. But high levels of insulin deplete vitamin E levels in the body, so people with Syndrome X or type II diabetes have higher needs for vitamin E.

New Research on Vitamin E and Diabetes

Over the last few years, a great deal of exciting research has focused on the positive effects of vitamin E in diabetes. One such study found that four weeks of supplementation with vitamin E (400 IU per day) decreased oxidative stress—an excess of free radicals—in both type I and type II diabetes.

To clarify, type I diabetes, known as insulin-dependent diabetes, is characterized by inefficient production of blood-sugar-lowering insulin. Type II (non-insulin-dependent) diabetes, on the other hand, involves adequate amounts of insulin (at least in the initial stages of the disease) but the insulin that's produced doesn't work efficiently. So, vitamin E protects against complications in both types.

Another study, reported in the *American Journal of Clinical Nutrition,* found that 250 IU of natural vitamin E (d-alpha-tocopherol) taken three times a day by patients with type I diabetes decreased the oxidation of blood fats, including LDL cholesterol, after only three months of supplementation. The benefits ended after the subjects stopped taking vitamin E, leading the researchers to recommend considering life-long supplementation with vitamin E in patients with type I diabetes. Still other studies have found that taking vitamin E might help reduce the risk of devel - oping diabetic retinopathy (damage to blood vessels of the retina) as well as the severe kidney problems associated with diabetes in type I patients.

Patients with type II diabetes can also benefit from taking vitamin E. As you will recall, limiting oxidation of LDL cholesterol is important for decreasing the risk of heart disease, and a study published in the journal *Diabetes Care* in 2000 found that 800 IU per day of vitamin E taken for four weeks decreased LDL oxidation, as well as another risk factor for heart attack, in patients with type II diabetes. These findings are very encouraging because people with diabetes have a higher-than-average risk of heart disease.

While vitamin E is extremely safe, some caution is required in diabetics. If you are taking insulin or hypoglycemic drugs, you may have to reduce the dosages of these drugs. This is because vitamin E will improve your health so you will need less of these drugs, and if you do not reduce the dosage, you could end up overdosing. However, it is very important that you adjust the dosage of vitamin E and the drugs in cooperation with your physician.

In addition, people with "leaky" blood vessels, found in some types of diabetic retinopathy (eye disease), could develop problems with vitamin E supplements, due to the nutrient's mild anticoagulant properties. While such problems are not common, caution is warranted.

Vitamin E Protects the Skin

Wrinkles are an age-related condition that develops over time, like Alzheimer's disease and heart disease. Vitamin E slows down the aging process, so it probably can help delay the appearance of wrinkles, especially when used as part of a comprehensive program to maintain youthful skin.

Many factors contribute to the formation and deepening of wrinkles, including exposure to environmental pollutants, poor nutrition, smoking, and, especially, too much time in the sun. The damaging effects of sunlight on the skin are cumulative, but they may not be obvious until years later.

A recent cell-culture study found that natural vitamin E protects skin by blocking the activity of protein kinase C. This enzyme promotes the breakdown of collagen, one of the main structural proteins of the skin. Aging and air pollution increase collagen breakdown, but it seems that vitamin E can protect against this.

The best approach to prevent wrinkles is to avoid exposure to cigarette smoke and pollutants, eat well, limit your time in the sun, and take antioxidants—such as vitamin E and vitamin C—that help protect against the damage from sunlight which ages the skin.

Vitamins E and C Protect against Sunburn

A recent study in the *Journal of the American Academy of Dermatology* found that taking vitamins C and E can help protect against sunburn. The vitamins do not accomplish this by acting as a sunscreen, but instead by enhancing the body's ability to withstand burning.

In the study, Bernadette Eberlein-Konig, M.D., and her colleagues from the dermatology clinic at the Technical University of Munich exposed twenty men and women to ultraviolet (UV) light. Then Eberlein-Konig gave half of the subjects either a placebo or supplements containing 2,000 mg of vitamin C and 1,000 IU of natural vitamin E daily for eight days, after which portions of the subjects' skin were again exposed to UV light. People taking vitamin C and E showed an increased resistance to sunburn while those taking the placebo showed an increased sensitivity to UV light.

"This study shows for the first time that systemic administration of vitamins C and E reduces the sunburn reaction in humans. . . Systemic photoprotection is convenient and could provide a desirable basic UV shield for the entire body surface," Eberlein-Konig wrote in the study.

In a study published in the *American Journal of Clinical Nutrition* in 2000, researchers reported that oral carotenoids and vitamin E protected against free radical damage to the skin from ultraviolet light. Benefits were greatest with the combination of carotenoids (25 mg total carotenoids per day) and natural vitamin E (335 mg, or 500 IU), as opposed to carotenoids alone.

Previous research has shown that topical applications of vitamins C and E have a weak sunblocking effect, so using vitamin E internally and externally (both as an oral supplement and as an ingredient in topical lotions) appears to be the best way to protect yourself from damaging UV rays when you do spend time in the sun.

Vitamin E's Benefits for Minor Cuts and More Serious Burns

Vitamin E might help heal minor cuts and burns, which are a lot like sunburns. In burns and cuts, free radicals flood the site of injury, causing inflammation and redness. These free radicals are supposed to prevent infection, but sometimes the body doesn't know when to turn them off. An ointment containing vitamin E should help the healing process and restore normal vitamin E levels in the skin. You can also pop vitamin E capsules with a needle and dab the oil on minor household burns and cuts after a scab has formed.

More severe burns generate very large quantities of free radicals, which can slow the healing process. It's easy to imagine the free radical generation that takes place on the damaged skin's surface in burn victims. But the damage doesn't end on the surface.

Free radicals can wreak havoc deeper in the body as a result of burns, damaging red blood cells, oxidizing fats and impairing the function of white blood cells called neutrophils. Neutrophils normally act as phagocytes, meaning they surround and engulf bacteria and other foreign invaders in the body, thereby protecting us from disease.

Neutrophils
White blood cells that surround and engulf bacteria and other foreign invaders in the body, protecting us from disease.

When neutrophils are impaired by free radicals (as in serious burns), our defenses against dangerous invaders are compromised. Vitamin E acts as a free radical scavenger to protect neutrophil function among human burn victims. In one recent study, oral vitamin E was also found to protect the heart in test animals suffering from burns by reducing heart inflammation that typically follows burn trauma.

Clearly, vitamin E can quench many of the free radicals that result from burns. However, if you're talking about topical use, the problem is more pragmatic: How do you apply vitamin E to a serious burn, when the burned person is likely to scream in pain? Carlson Laboratories (1-800-323-4141), which has the broadest and perhaps most reputable selection of natural vitamin E products, sells a vitamin E spray that can be helpful in such cases.

Evan Shute, M.D., who pioneered the clinical use of vitamin E in heart disease, felt that his lasting contribution to medicine would be the use of vitamin E in treating burns. Shute treated many burn victims with vitamin E, and it consistently promoted healing and minimized scarring. If you have a burn, you're likely to get benefits by both taking the vitamin orally and applying it topically.

Vitamin E Protects against Damage from Exercise

Few people realize it, but aerobic activity, including aerobics, cross-country skiing, running and more, increases the production of free radicals, which can damage muscle tissue and result in inflammation, aching muscles, and a feeling of being wiped out. But vitamin E acts like a sponge, soaking up those free radicals before they damage tissues.

In a study by German researchers, regular exercise increased the levels of DNA damage in human subjects. However, when these subjects took vitamin E supplements, the exercise-induced DNA damage was virtually eliminated. According to Lester Packer, Ph.D., a researcher at the University of California, Berkeley, and one of the foremost authorities on antioxidants, vitamin E can probably reduce exercise-induced fatigue. Quicker recovery from fatigue should, in turn, improve exercise performance.

Also, research published in the journal *Nutrition* in 1999 reported that marathon runners who took 1000 IU of vitamin E daily for two weeks before a race had fewer cases of abdominal pain and less occurrence of blood in their stools (which indicates gastrointestinal bleeding) than runners in the placebo group. This type of pain and bleeding is common in marathon runners, so vitamin E might help this group in a major way.

It may seem counterintuitive that exercise—something so good for your health—actually increases the production of nasty free radicals. This doesn't mean you should become a couch potato; instead, simply add vitamin E supplements to your workout regimen.

The List of Benefits Goes On

Vitamin E protects against still more health hazards—for example, secondhand smoke. Cigarette smoke—like other forms of air pollution—increases a person's free radical burden. Even if you don't smoke, it could be a problem. Nonsmoking spouses of smokers are 3.5 times more likely to develop lung cancer, compared to people living in smoke-free houses. Breathing cigarette smoke passively is comparable to smoking anywhere from one to ten cigarettes yourself daily.

When a nonsmoker breathes in smoke from a spouse, friend, or coworker, the many pollutants and cancer-causing chemicals in tobacco smoke attack the membranes and DNA of his or her body's cells. If you live or work with a smoker, you are in effect a smoker. Vitamin E can help reduce the damage. So can opening the window.

Vitamin E also protects lung function. In a study of 178 men and women, it was found that those who consumed the most vitamin E had significantly better lung function than those who consumed the least amount. And vitamin E protects red blood cells from damage. Without enough vitamin E, red blood cells die sooner than they should. Adequate vitamin E, therefore, is needed to prevent hemolytic anemia, and the depression and lethargy that usually accompany this condition.

Vitamin E is not a panacea (or cure-all), but it plays numerous roles in health, so it's not entirely surprising that vitamin E benefits a wide range of different conditions. Every cell in the body requires vitamin E, which is why the nutrient benefits cells as different as heart and brain cells. Vitamin E also plays important roles in promoting the normal behavior of genes, and genes contain the most basic biological instructions for the body. When Drs. Evan and Wilfrid Shute were using vitamin E in the 1940s and 1950s, many of their critics said the vitamin seemed like a panacea. What they were lacking was an explanation of why vitamin E works. Today, we have that explanation, and time has largely proved the Shutes right about vitamin E and its many benefits.

CHAPTER 7

WHAT YOU SHOULD KNOW ABOUT TOCOTRIENOLS

Vitamin E comes in eight forms and two groups: four of them are tocopherols and four are tocotrienols. Among the tocopherols are alpha-tocopherol, beta-tocopherol, delta-tocopherol and gamma-tocopherol. Likewise, the tocotrienols include alpha-, beta-, delta- and gamma-tocotrienol. All eight forms are still vitamin E, but they each have slightly different chemical structures and actions in the body.

This chapter will fill you in on the tocotrienol forms of vitamin E. As you'll discover, they have some impressive benefits that scientists are just beginning to understand. The next chapter will help you decide what types of vitamin E supplements to buy.

Tocotrienols Offer Antioxidant Activity and Heart-Protective Benefits

Tocotrienols are relatively new on the scene, but some research has shown they have impressive antioxidant activity. Tocotrienols are not as bioavailable (well absorbed) by the body after oral supplementation as tocopherols are. They do, however, penetrate the skin quickly and efficiently,

Tocotrienols
A group of four forms of vitamin E that differ slightly from tocopherols in their structure and function in the body.

fighting excessive free radicals produced from ultraviolet rays or ozone.

Like alpha-tocopherol, tocotrienols may be beneficial in protecting against heart disease. One way they do this is by inhibiting LDL oxidation. Tocotrienols are also noted for their ability to lower cholesterol and reduce inflammation, according to a study published in the *Journal of Nutrition* in 2001. These actions might interfere with the formation of atherosclerotic plaque—or might reduce the size of existing lesions—which, you'll remember, can block blood flow and lead to heart attacks.

Lesion
An abnormal growth of cells, such as those involved in forming "cholesterol deposits."

In the study cited above, mice with atherosclerotic lesions that were fed the tocotrienol-rich fraction of rice bran had a 42 percent decrease in the size of their lesions, whereas mice supplemented with alpha-tocopherol experienced only an 11 percent reduction in lesions. The tocotrienols did decrease levels of cholesterol and triglyceride (another blood lipid), but the greater improvement in lesions led the researchers to conclude that tocotrienols were superior to alpha-tocopherol in minimizing such lesions. The tocotrienol content of rice bran oil—which has cholesterol-lowering activity in humans—might help explain the purported heart benefits of this oil over other vegetable oils.

Encouraging Early Research for Fighting Breast Cancer

In recent research, tocotrienols have shown promise in fighting breast cancer cells. When the mammary cancer cells of mice were studied in culture, tocotrienols were more effective than tocopherols at inducing apoptosis, or cell death, of the cancer cells. Results with human breast cancer cells have also been promising.

In a study reported in the journal *Nutrition and Cancer,* alpha-, gamma-, and delta-tocotrienols caused cell death in human breast cancer cells in culture. Of the four tocopherols, only delta-tocopherol induced cell death in the cancer cells. The researchers concluded that naturally-occuring tocotrienols and natural delta-tocopherol are effective at inducing cell death in human breast cancer cells. A recent animal study found that tocotrienols even increased the benefits of drugs, such as tamoxifen, which fight breast cancer.

Relative to the research on alpha-tocopherol, the research on tocotrienols is still in its infancy, and the research on tocotrienols does not mean they are a treatment or a cure for breast cancer. More human studies are needed to find out how, and in what amounts, tocotrienols can benefit cancer, heart health and perhaps other conditions. However, the future looks bright for these previously underestimated forms of vitamin E.

Weighing Supplementation with Tocotrienols and Tocopherols

It's important to remember that all eight forms of vitamin E—not just alpha-tocopherol and not just the tocotrienols—are likely important to good health. The intriguing new research on toco - trienols doesn't prove that these types of vitamin E are preferable to alpha-tocopherol for all purposes. Rather, it points out the importance of the full spectrum of benefits from the whole family of vitamin E forms.

There are probably other advantages to taking both tocopherols and tocotrienols that have not yet been researched in depth. As we learn more about them, we may discover new benefits of the tocotrienols, not just as a group, but as four individual kinds of tocotrienols. In the meantime, look for "mixed tocotrienols" and "mixed toco- pherols" on vitamin labels if you want to take advantage of the whole range of vitamin E bene- fits. More and more companies are incorporating a broader array of vitamin E forms into multi- vitamins.

Unlike alpha-tocopherol, tocotrienols (and the other three tocopherols) are only available from natural sources. That means, when comparing labels on supplement bottles, you don't have to worry about trying to tell the difference between the superior natural forms and the inferior syn- thetic vitamin E that you want to avoid. Whatever products you choose, be sure to check the expi- ration dates and to store your vitamin E in a cool, dry place away from any light, instead of in the often warm and humid bathroom medicine cabi- net. In the next chapter, we'll explain everything you need to know about buying natural vitamin E products.

CHAPTER 8

SHOPPING FOR AND TAKING VITAMIN E

By now, you should appreciate the health benefits of vitamin E. One of the best things you can do for your health is to begin taking vitamin E supplements, if you aren't already. While doing so might seem as simple as buying a bottle of vitamin E, finding a quality product can often be difficult and confusing. In this chapter, we explain the important differences between natural and synthetic vitamin E and the many different forms of this vitamin. We also offer a number of tips to help you choose among the many different types of vitamin E supplements.

Vitamin E—A Fat-Soluble Vitamin We Need

Vitamin E is an essential nutrient. It is a fat-soluble vitamin (in contrast to water-soluble nutrients like vitamin C) which means that it functions primarily in the fatty portions of cells. It also means that vitamin E supplements are best taken with a little fat or oil (as is usually found in a regular meal) for optimal absorption.

Fat-soluble Vitamin

A vitamin that dissolves only in oil and is found in the fatty parts of food. Fat-soluble vitamins like vitamin E are best absorbed when con-sumed with a small amount of fat.

The Recommended Dietary Allowance is 15

mg or 22 IU daily for an adult. However, the average American gets only about 8 IU from his diet. Furthermore, vitamin E requirements increase with a higher intake of polyunsaturated fatty acids (PUFAs)—the types of fats used in fried foods and salad dressings. Americans generally eat so many PUFAs that they need to compensate for the damaging effects of these fats.

Vegetable oils are high in PUFAs, and vitamin E requirements increase when a person consumes a lot of PUFAs. Vitamin E is needed to prevent PUFAs from oxidizing, or turning rancid. For example, anyone eating fried chicken and french fries several times a week is consuming a huge quantity of PUFAs and will need a lot more vitamin E than would, say, someone who chooses not to eat any fried foods. In fact, researchers have found that 120 IU of vitamin E supplementation daily greatly reduced DNA damage among men eating a diet high in PUFAs. Of course, it's better to avoid or strictly limit your intake of these oils and fried foods, instead of simply taking extra vitamin E.

There's also a misconception that common vegetable oils, such as peanut or soybean oil, are good dietary sources of vitamin E. Such oils tend to be very high in the gamma-tocopherol form of vitamin E, not the alpha-tocopherol form. (Tocopherol is the chemical term to describe one form of vitamin E, and the alpha-tocopherol fraction of the vitamin E molecule is the most active one in the human body.) Although gamma-tocopherol has some antioxidant properties, the body primarily needs the alpha-tocopherol form of vitamin E. It's possible that consuming of a lot of vegetable oils containing gamma-tocopherol interferes with the body's use of alpha-tocopherol.

Once again, it's important to understand that

you should avoid vegetable oils (including corn, cottonseed, safflower, soybean, and sunflower oils and products made with these oils) *and* take vitamin E supplements. Doing both are critical steps for dramatically improving your health. The vitamin E protects the good oils (such as omega-3 fish oils) that should be part of your diet, and it also reduces lung damage from air pollution, a sad fact of modern life.

Eight Is Enough

Many vitamins have only one form, but—as we explained in the last chapter—vitamin E actually has eight. While keeping them straight can be a little confusing, it's important to realize that all of the various forms of vitamin E are probably important for health.

d-alpha-tocopherol
The most abundant form of vitamin E in our bodies and in vitamin supplements.

As we've mentioned throughout this book, alpha-tocopherol is the most common form of vit-amin E, both in our bodies and in vitamin supplements. And, as you'll recall from earlier chapters, vitamin E was first recognized for its importance in reproduction. Alpha-tocopherol is the form of vitamin E most strongly associated with that function and so it has garnered the most attention over the years.

But the other seven other forms of vitamin E are important, too. You'll recall that the eight forms of vitamin E are divided into four toco-trienols and four tocopherols. These two groups have slightly different chemical structures and functions in the body.

Choose Natural Vitamin E over Synthetic

The most important thing to know is that natural

International Unit (IU)

A unit of weight usually used for fat-soluble vitamins. For example, 1.49 IU and 1 mg are the same amount of natural vitamin E.

forms of vitamin E are far better than synthetic forms. For years, researchers believed that natural vitamin E was 1.36 times more potent than synthetic vitamin E when measured in milligrams (mg). This difference was found in animal studies, and because of it, the international unit (IU) standard was developed to equalize natural and synthetic vitamin E. However, there are still major differences between natural and synthetic.

In recent human studies, Graham Burton, Ph.D., and Robert Acuff, Ph.D., found that natural vitamin E was absorbed and retained twice as well as synthetic vitamin E. Basically, when people were given equal amounts of natural and synthetic vitamin E, the levels of natural vitamin E rose twice as high in the bloodstream and in tissues. The reason, according to a number of researchers, is that the human body opts for the natural molecule over the synthetic replicas. This means that, even using the IU standard, the natural vitamin E is better absorbed—and the synthetic falls way short. Buying natural vitamin E, therefore, gives you much more value for your money.

Natural Vitamin E

Forms of vitamin E that are derived from natural sources (such as soybeans) and that are absorbed and retained best by the body.

It's easy to distinguish synthetic from natural vitamin E, but you have to read the fine print on the label. Natural vitamin E is identified as "d-alpha-" tocopherol, whereas the synthetic is "dl-alpha-" tocopherol. A good way to remember the difference is that your body doesn't like the synthetic form (dl-alpha-tocopherol) as much as the natural form. Conversely, the natural form, or d-alpha-tocopherol, is delicious to your body.

Fortunately, you only have to worry about looking for the "d" when it comes to alpha-tocopherol. That's because the other seven forms of vitamin E are only available in natural forms. Unfortunately, not all labels specify whether the alpha-tocopherol is from natural or synthetic sources. If it doesn't say it's natural (that is, there's no "d"), assume it's synthetic. Natural vitamin E will be more expensive than synthetic, but you get what you pay for. And, relatively speaking, purchasing natural vitamin E is a wise investment in your health.

Natural Forms and Esterification

When choosing a vitamin E supplement that's best for you, it's important to understand about the various types of vitamin E typically found in supplements. As explained above, d-alpha-tocopherol is the most biologically active among the different types of vitamin E. It is a natural

Esterification
The process of combining an acid with an alcohol (as with alpha-tocopheryl-acetate) to increase stability and decrease oxidation.

and highly absorbable form of vitamin E. Its only drawback is a relatively limited shelf life, though it is stable for at least three years, provided it is stored in a cool, dry environment.

Another natural form of vitamin E, d-alpha-tocopheryl acetate, is more stable in terms of shelf life. The acetate means it has been ester-ified—essentially combined with an acid—to improve stability and shelf life. Without esterifi-cation, alpha-tocopherol is prone to oxidation. Once it is oxidized, vitamin E doesn't do us much good. D-alpha tocopheryl acetate is probably the best form for people actively trying to prevent heart disease, because it has been used in many medical studies.

Esterification is especially important in multivitamins and cosmetic products containing forms of vitamin E, since exposure to air and interacting with other ingredients can oxidize the vitamin E. Combining alpha-tocopherol with these acids is safe and it protects the vitamin E from damage.

Another esterified form of vitamin E, d-alpha-tocopheryl succinate, which we discussed in Chapter 2, is also a stable form of natural vitamin E. The most promising studies on vitamin E's anti-cancer properties have tended to use this particular form.

Natural Mixed Tocopherols
The four tocopherol forms of vitamin E that occur naturally in foods, including d-alpha-, d-beta-, d-gamma- and d-delta-tocopherol.

A more "naturelike" approach to taking vitamin E is to seek out a "mixed tocopherol" product. This type of product contains a specific amount of natural d-alpha-tocopherol (usually 400 IU), plus a small amount of natural beta-, gamma-, and delta-tocopherols. Although alpha-tocopherol is considered the most biologically active form of vitamin E, the other fractions also have antioxidant properties and are believed to be of some benefit.

Finding the Best Form for You

The best form of vitamin E varies according to the individual. Each of the natural forms of vitamin E is good, though they have slightly different properties. After understanding the merits and drawbacks of each type (as we explained above), you should evaluate which type is best for you based on what diseases you're most at risk for and what you eat.

It's important to know that all four types of tocopherols are found in natural foods, but d-alpha-tocopherol is the one that gets stripped away the most in processed vegetable oils. If you eat a lot of "fast" and convenience foods, supplementing your diet with d-alpha-tocopherol can partly compensate for some of what you're missing in your diet. But again, it would be far better to avoid processed vegetable oils and convenience and "fast" foods in the first place.

If you eat a lot of unprocessed, nutrient-dense, natural foods (which you should strive to do for better health), a mixed natural tocopherol supplement is probably a better choice because it more closely reproduces how vitamin E occurs in nature, with all four tocopherols. For disease prevention, our personal preference is a "mixed natural tocopherol" vitamin E supplement. Most natural vitamin E supplements, by the way, are produced from soybeans.

400 IU—The Standard Dose for Most People

In general, most adults would do well taking 400 IU daily of natural vitamin E. This dosage reduces the oxidation of cholesterol and, based on human studies, leads to dramatic reductions in the incidence of coronary heart disease. Higher doses can further reduce the oxidation of cholesterol, but it might be better to take a combination of antioxidants than to take very high doses of vitamin E.

Antioxidants work as a team of synergistic nutrients. So as good as vitamin E is, a combination of antioxidants is preferable. Consider taking 400 IU of vitamin E, 1,000 mg or more of vitamin C, 15,000–25,000 IU of mixed carotenoids, 30 mg of coenzyme Q_{10}, and 50 mg of alpha-lipoic acid. Many "antioxidant formulas" contain these and other antioxidants and enable you to simplify the number of tablets or capsules you take.

Every adult should probably be taking vitamin E supplements. People who live in very polluted cities, or those who eat large amounts of fried foods or vegetable oils, exercise strenuously, or live in high altitudes should probably take at least 400 IU daily, even if they are currently healthy. Children should also take vitamin E, but the dosage should be adjusted to their weight.

The Safety of Vitamin E

In general, vitamin E is exceptionally safe. Clinical trials of vitamin E supplementation at daily doses as high as 3,200 IU in a wide variety of people for up to two years have not shown any unfavorable side effects.

There are some risks you should be aware of, however. Although vitamin E reduces the risk of heart disease and thrombotic stroke (caused by blood clots), it slightly increases the risk of hemorrhagic stroke (caused by leaky blood vessels). The risk, in general, is insignificant because the vast majority of strokes are caused by blood clots, which vitamin E can help prevent.

Along this line, some research has shown that vitamin E supplements might amplify the effects of prescription anticoagulant (or blood-thinning) drugs. However, other research has shown that vitamin E does not have this effect. We suspect the varying effects may be dose-related. If you're taking aspirin *and* a prescription anticoagulant *and* vitamin E, all these anticoagulants may be a bit too much. If you are taking an anticoagulant drug, discuss your desire to take vitamin E with your physician.

People with diabetes who take vitamin E may have to adjust their dosage of insulin or hypo-glycemic drugs—this is a good sign, indicating a lessening of diabetic symptoms. And people with rheumatic heart disease, in which half the heart is damaged, should start taking only 50–100 IU of vitamin E under a physician's supervision. The rea-son is, the stronger part of the heart may respond to vitamin E much faster than the weaker part.

Vitamin E Works Slowly but Surely

Occasionally people will experience quick relief from something like sore breasts by taking vita-min E—or they'll see evidence of cuts and burns healing faster. But most often vitamin E just works subtly and preventively, helping to slow the aging process and prevent degenerative diseases. On a day-to-day basis, you probably won't notice that your body has fewer damaging free radicals but your risk of disease will lessen over the long term because of this benefit. The longer you take vita-min E, the more you'll probably find you're in bet-ter health than other people your age who don't take vitamin E.

Taking vitamin E supplements can significantly lower your risk of heart disease, enhance the func-tioning of your immune system, and likely reduce your risk of developing Alzheimer's disease. Vita-min E, however, is not a magic bullet or panacea. You can't simply take a pill and expect to gain per-fect health. The other components of a lifestyle that promotes health include eating a diet rich in protein and fruits and vegetables, exercising moderately (at least going for a walk several times a week), and managing psychological stresses. Vitamin E supplements, in combination with a general antioxidant formula or multivitamin, can provide many health benefits—and increase your likelihood of having a long, functional, and satisfying life.

CONCLUSION

Vitamin E is the main antioxidant that protects all cells from damage, so it's one of the most important nutrient supplements you can take to keep your whole body healthy and avoid disease. As you've learned, vitamin E helps protect against leading killers, including Alzheimer's disease, cancer, and heart disease. It enhances the immune system, bolstering the body's defenses against colds and other infections. Vitamin E also slows the aging process, probably delaying the onset of such conditions as cataracts and wrinkles. And it helps heal or alleviate many minor health complaints—including everything from burns to menopausal hot flashes.

If you didn't pay much attention to vitamin E until reading this book, you're probably amazed at just how much of a health protector vitamin E really is. Research on the many benefits of vitamin E continues to pile up at a furious pace and these benefits impress virtually everyone, from once-skeptical doctors to questioning health reporters.

To tap the potential of all vitamin E's benefits, though, you must take supplements of the nutrient. You simply can't get enough vitamin E for therapeutic effects from foods alone.

Numerous supplements receive a lot of hype these days and many deliver on their promises. Vitamin E, though, is one that has stood the test of time in both scientific research and clinical practice. It's a tried-and-true nutritional supplement that should be a part of everyone's supplement regimen for better health.

In sum, do as we do: weigh the evidence, and take vitamin E supplements.

SELECTED
REFERENCES

Boaz, M, Smetana, S, Weinstein, T, et al. Secondary prevention with antioxidants of cardiovascular disease in endstage renal disease (SPACE): randomised placebo-controlled trial. *Lancet*, 2000; 356:1213–1218.

Bursell, SE, Clermont, C, Aiello, LP, et al. High-dose vitamin E supplementation normalizes retinal blood flow and creatinine clearance in patients with type I diabetes. *Diabetes Care*, 1999; 22: 1245–1251.

Burton, GW, Traber, MG, Acuff, RV, et al. Human plasma and tissue a-tocopherol concentrations in response to supplementation with deuterated natural and synthetic vitamin E. *American Journal of Clinical Nutrition*, 1998; 67:669–684.

Eberlein-König, B, Placzek, M, Pryzybilla, B. Protective effect against sunburn of combined systemic ascorbic acid (vitamin C) and d-a-tocopherol (vitamin E). *Journal of the American Academy of Dermatology*, 1998; 38:45–48.

Engelen, W, Keenoy, BM, Vertommen, J, De Leeuw, I. Effects of long-term supplementation with moderate pharmacologic doses of vitamin E are saturable and reversible in patients with type I diabetes. *American Journal of Clinical Nutrition*, 2000; 72(5)1142–1149.

Grundman, M. Vitamin E and Alzheimer disease: the basis for additional clinical trials. *American Journal of Clinical Nutrition,* 2000; 71: 630S–636S.

Heinonen, OP, Albanes, D, Virtano, J, et al. Prostate cancer and supplementation with a-tocopherol and b-carotene: incidence and mortality in a controlled trial. *Journal of the National Cancer Institute,* 1998; 90:440–446.

Ishi, K, et al. Prevention of mammary tumorigenesis in acatalasemic mice by vitamin E supplementation. *Japanese Journal of Cancer Research,* 1996; 87:680–684.

Jialal, I, Traber, M, Deveraj, S. Is there a vitamin E paradox? *Current Opinion in Lipidology,* 2001; 12:49–53.

Katz, DL, Hawaz, H, Boukhalil, J, et al. Acute effects of oats and vitamin E on endothelial responses to ingested fat. *American Journal of Preventive Medicine,* 2001; 20:124–129.

Kaul, N, Devaraj, S, Jialal, I. Alpha-tocopherol and atherosclerosis. *Experimental Biology and Medicine,* 2001; 226(1):5–12.

Kodama, H, Yamaguchi, R, Fukuda, J, et al. Increased oxidative deoxyribonucleic acid damage in the spermatozoa of infertile male patients. *Fertility and Sterility,* 1997; 68:519–524.

Meydani, S, Meydani, M, et al. Vitamin E supplementation and in vivo immune response in healthy elderly subjects. *Journal of the American Medical Association,* 1997; 27:1380–1386.

Miller, JW. Vitamin E and memory: is it vascular protection? *Nutrition Reviews,* 2000; 58:109–111.

Packer, L. Oxidants, antioxidant nutrients and the athlete. *Journal of Sports Sciences,* 1997; 15: 353–363.

Plotnick, GD, Corretti, MC, Vogel, RA. Effect of antioxidant vitamins on the transient impairment of endothelium-dependent brachial artery vasoactivity following a single high-fat meal. *JAMA,* 1997; 278:1682–1686.

Poulin, JE, Cover, C, Gustafson, MR, Kay, MB. Vitamin E prevents oxidative modification of brain and lymphocyte band 3 proteins during aging. *Proceedings of the National Academy of Sciences,* 1996; 93:5600–3.

Qureshi, AA, Salser, WA, Parmar, R, Emeson, EE. Novel tocotrienols of rice bran inhibit atherosclerotic lesions in C57BL/6 ApoE-deficient mice. *Journal of Nutrition,* 2001; 131(10):2606–2618.

Rimm, EB, et al. Vitamin E consumption and the risk of coronary heart disease in men. *New England Journal of Medicine,* 1993; 328:1450–1456.

Sano, M, Ernesto, C, Thomas, RG, et al. A controlled trial of selegiline, alpha-tocopherol, or both as treatment for Alzheimer's disease. *The New England Journal of Medicine,* 1997; 336: 1216–1222.

Seth, RK, Kharb, S. Protective function of alpha-tocopherol against the process of cataractogenesis in humans. *Annals of Nutrition and Metabolism,* 1999; 43:286–289.

Stampfer, MJ, et al. Vitamin E consumption and the risk of coronary heart disease in women. *New England Journal of Medicine,* 1993; 328: 1444–1449.

Stephens, NG, Parsons, A, Schofield, PM, et al. Randomised controlled trial of vitamin E in patients with coronary disease: Cambridge Heart Antioxidant Study (CHAOS). *Lancet,* 1996; 347: 781–786.

Verlangieri, A. Effects of a-tocopherol supplementation on experimentally induced primate atherosclerosis. *Journal of American College of Nutrition,* 1992; 11:130–137.

OTHER BOOKS
AND RESOURCES

Challem, J, Berkson, B, and Smith, MD. *Syndrome X: The Complete Nutritional Program to Prevent and Reverse Insulin Resistance.* New York, NY: John Wiley & Sons, 2000.

Challem, J, and Brown, L. *User's Guide to Vitamins and Minerals.* North Bergen, NJ: Basic Health Publications, 2002.

Challem, J, and Dolby, V. *Homocysteine: The Secret Killer.* New Canaan, CT: Keats Publishing, 1997.

Murray, Michael, and Pizzorno, Joseph. *Encyclopedia of Natural Medicine,* revised second edition. Prima Publishing: Rocklin, CA, 1998.

Smith, MD. *Going Against the Grain.* Chicago, IL: Contemporary Publishing, 2002.

Smith, MD. *User's Guide to Chromium.* North Bergen, NJ: Basic Health Publications, 2002.

GreatLife Magazine
Consumer magazine with articles on vitamins, minerals, herbs, and foods.
Available for free at many health and natural food stores.

Let's Live Magazine

Consumer magazine with emphasis on the health benefits of vitamins, minerals, and herbs.

Customer service:
1-800-676-4333
P.O. Box 74908
Los Angeles, CA 90004

Subscriptions: 12 issues per year, $19.95 in the U.S.; $31.95 outside the U.S.

The Nutrition Reporter™ newsletter

Monthly newsletter that summarizes recent medical research on vitamins, minerals, and herbs.

Customer service:
P.O. Box 30246
Tucson, AZ 85751-0246
e-mail: jack@thenutritionreporter.com
www.nutritionreporter.com

Subscriptions: $26 per year (12 issues) in the U.S.; $32 U.S. or $48 CNC for Canada; $38 for other countries

Physical Magazine

Magazine oriented to body builders and other serious athletes.

Customer service:
1-800-676-4333
P.O. Box 74908
Los Angeles, CA 90004

Subscriptions: 12 issues per year, $19.95 in the U.S.; $31.95 outside the U.S.

Centers for Disease Control and Prevention (CDC)

http://www.cdc.gov/

Learn about a wide range of diseases at this government website.

MEDLINE
http://www.ncbi.nlm.nih.gov/entrez/query
For specific medical journal abstracts.

National Center for Complementary and Alternative Medicine, National Institutes of Health (NIH)
http://nccam.nih.gov/nccam/
Search a database of 180,000 bibliographic citations regarding complementary and alternative therapies extracted from MEDLINE.

Office of Dietary Supplements, National Institutes of Health
http://dietary-supplements.info.nih.gov/
Scientific resources (including recent research findings regarding supplements), general information about supplements, and programs and activities of the Office of Dietary Supplements.

Vitamin E Research and Information Service (VERIS)
http://www.veris-online.org
Read abstracts of antioxidant research.

INDEX